Candida Cleanse: Cure Candida Naturally in 14 Days

Contents

Introduction

Thank you for downloading this book, *"Candida Cleanse: Cure Candida in 14 Days Naturally"*.

In this book, you will learn about Candida Albicans infection and how you can treat it naturally. This book gives more information on how you can go about with the strict Candida diet and cleansing process.

I hope that you learn a lot from this book.

Again, thank you.

Enjoy!

Chapter 1 – Candida Albicans

Overview

Candida Albicans is a kind of fungi (or form of yeast) that is normally found on the skin and in mucous membranes like the mouth, vagina, and rectum. The fungus can travel through the blood stream and can affect internal organs, including the heart.

Candida Albicans is part of the gut flora, which is a group of microorganisms that inhabits your intestine and your mouth. Almost all humans have it but it only becomes an infectious agent when there are changes in the body's environment that cause its rapid replication. When the population begins to get out of control, it can cause the weakening of the intestinal wall. When it penetrates the bloodstream, it will release toxic byproducts into the body.

These toxic byproducts will cause damage not just in your organs but also on tissue cells and the immune system. Its major waste product is Acetaldehyde, identified as a poisonous toxin that promotes free radical activities in the body. The liver also converts Acetaldehyde into ethanol or drinking alcohol. There are some people who report to have feelings of drunkenness. Some even complain of a hangover even without drinking alcohol the night before. People with Candida Albicans complain of debilitating fatigue, this is due to the high levels of ethanol in their system.

Causes

Most of the time, infections occur for no apparent reason. One of the most common probable causes could be the use of antibiotics that destroy both the healthy and harmful microorganisms found in the body which causes the rapid growth of Candida. The condition is referred to as *Candidiasis Moniliasis* or simply, a yeast infection.

Candidiasis Moniliasis is referred to as "thrush" when it grows in the mouth, and it is more common in infants. The infection is manifested on the skin as inflamed, red, and almost scaly rash, similar to a diaper rash.

When it occurs in the vagina, it is "vaginalitis moniliasis" or a yeast infection. When it occurs in the nails, it is called "candidal onchomycosis". The digestive tract and the esophagus can also have yeast infection.

The infection in the penis is more common in men who are uncircumcised than men who are. Men can also get infected during sexual intercourse, when their partner has the infection.

Symptoms

Thrush appears like a creamy-white or bluish-white patches that are visible on the tongue, which appears to be inflamed. The patches can also take on a red discoloration along the lining of the mouth or the throat.

When there is vaginatis, a yellowish-white discharge appears. The walls of the vagina and the vulva (the external genital area) are inflamed, causing excessive itching and burning feeling.

The infection on the fingernails or the toenails is characterized by a painful swelling around the nail. The area has red discoloration and pus is likely to develop.

When there is inflammation in the penis, the head is usually inflamed.

When the infection reaches the bloodstream, the internal organs are put at risk, including the heart, kidneys, lungs, brain, and the eyes. Symptoms include:

- Heart: murmurs and heart valve damage
- Kidneys: presence of blood in the urine
- Lungs: presence of bloody sputum
- Brain: seizures and extreme changes in behavior
- Eyes: blurred vision and pain

Other symptoms that can be related to the presence of Candida Albicans infection are:

- Migraine
- Poor memory
- Poor concentration
- Depression
- Fatigue
- Irritability
- Bloating
- Sensitivity to strong odors
- Allergy
- Recurrent sore throat
- Heartburn
- Diarrhea
- Numbness
- Weak muscles
- Tingling sensations
- Toe nail fungus
- Athlete's foot

Candida Albicans Infection Risk Factors

Candidiasis is not a condition that is acquired from an external source that can be easily remedied by the use of medications. It is the result of one's lifestyle, eating habits, environmental source, and even emotional influences that lead to decreased biological functionality for the body. This is because Candida Albicans is naturally occurring in the body, thus, anyone can develop the infection.

Yeast and other harmful microorganisms will not replicate and mutate into pathogenic forms unless the conditions favor their growth and proliferation are present.

Since Candida is naturally-occurring, it can be found in the natural microbial ecology of a healthy intestinal environment. When occurring in healthy concentrations, the main function of Candida is to feed on unfriendly microbes in the gut. When the healthy environment is destroyed, Candida yeast organisms will begin the mutation process into harmful fungus. The fungal organisms become powerful toxins, thus causing the signs and symptoms.

The damage in the intestinal walls will make the intestine more permeable substances that are normally blocked from entering the bloodstream through the intestinal lining.

Possible influences that can predispose you to developing Candida Albicans overgrowth:

- Improper pre-natal and infant nutrition
- Insufficient breast milk for the infant's consumption after birth
- Use of antibiotics
- Unhealthy diet
- Excessive consumption of alcohol
- Lack of sleep
- Lack of exercise
- Stress
- Having a sexual partner with infection

Find out more about Candida overgrowth in the next chapter.

Chapter 2 – Candida Overgrowth

What Is Candida Overgrowth?

Candida Albicans is present in the body because it has a role to perform. It is responsible in aiding the digestive tract and helps in the absorption of nutrients. It was discussed that Candida Albicans is naturally present in the body. Under normal and healthy conditions, it stays in the body without disturbing the system, as long as the acceptable amount is maintained. However, if the Candida organisms grow out of control and quickly multiply, your system would be at risk of infection.

Key Symptoms

Increase sugar craving is one of the most recognizable symptoms of Candida Albicans infection. There is also the increase in your body's susceptibility to the side effects of medications.

Sinusitis and recurrent colds are additional symptoms. Recurrent skin rashes also indicate that you have developed Candida Albicans infection.

In women, premenstrual syndrome is a common indication of an increase in the Candida organisms. There is also an evident decrease in sex drive. Pain is also felt, especially during intercourse. In men, the infection is indicated with bladder and prostate infections.

How Is It Diagnosed?

Doctors perform the following to rule out other possible illnesses that cause symptoms similar to Candida infection:

- *Blood test* – Your doctor would need to check the levels of IgG, IgA, and IgM candida antibodies in your blood. There are several laboratory tests that should be done. Having high levels of these antibodies would mean the occurrence of an overgrowth in Candida organisms.

- *Stool testing* – Most doctors agree that stool exam yields the most accurate results. A stool test will help determine if there are high levels of Candida Albicans in the color or the lower intestines. Through stool exam, the species of the yeast and corresponding treatment can be determined.

- *Urine organix dysbosis test* – This test helps detect the presence of D-Arabinitol, the most common waste product of Candida overgrowth. Elevation of Candida in the urine, mean that you have Candida overgrowth. This will also establish the occurrence of Candida in the upper gut and/or smaller intestines.

In ruling out the presence or the absence of Candida Albicans infection, and if the infection won't just go away and begins to involve other parts of the body, there are more extensive medical tests to be done:

- *Gynecologic exam* – To effectively diagnose vaginal yeast infection, doctors perform a full gynecologic exam. Tests include a speculum exam. A swab will be taken to test the discharge and an internal example will be performed, as well. A urine exam will try to establish the presence of blood.

- *Mouth (or skin) exam* – A quick mouth or skin exam is performed to confirm the presence of candidiasis.

Chapter 3 – When to Seek Professional Help for Candida Infection

When do you see a doctor?

It's simple, since you have already been presented with the common signs and symptoms of the medical condition; if you suspect that you have the infection, go to your doctor so that you will be properly diagnosed and given the appropriate medications and treatments. Do not immediately opt to do self-treatment without making sure that the symptoms indicate the presence of Candida Albicans infection.

However, there are those who resort to self-medication without getting the right diagnosis to what actually ails them. You have to take note that the symptoms mentioned above are quite common; hence, it is important that you get proper assessment. Plus, if you self-medicate, you might make the infection worse more than help treat it.

For women, if you are having abnormal vaginal discharge and you are not sure if you have yeast infection or other disease, you have to consult your doctor immediately.

Oral thrush would require medication and regular visits to your doctor. Since oral thrust is most common in children, it is imperative that you take your child to the doctor once you notice the visible manifestation of the symptoms. There is a possibility that you don't have Candida Albicans but you might be positive in other ailments.

When you feel that you fatigued all the time and lack the energy to get you through the day, you'll to go to your doctor. Fatigue can mean a lot of different types of ailments so you need to get immediate medical consultation so that you can make adjustments and work around whatever limitations you have.

Do you need to go to the hospital at once?

In most cases. The infection cannot be treated even if you are confined in the hospital. The increased levels of Candida Albicans in the bloodstream are enough to make you want to seek treatment.

Women who experience chills and fever, accompanied by nausea and vomiting, or when vaginal discharge is coupled with abdominal pain, it is imperative that they see a doctor or be tested as soon as possible. These symptoms also indicate that

Treating the Symptoms

Over-the-counter medications are usually prescribed to treat the physical manifestation of the symptoms. However, the effective treatment of Candida infection goes to the root cause of the problem, to stop yeast overgrowth. It is important to restore the "friendly" bacteria that keep tab of the presence of Candida organisms in your system. Your gut should also be zeroed in so that Candida can no longer enter the bloodstream.

You get rid of the yeast overgrowth by primarily changing your diet. For instance, sugar has to be eliminated because sugar feeds yeast, so if you have excessive sugar in your system, overgrowth is not impossible.

There other natural treatments that are recommended even by doctors to help treat Candida infection. The main goal is to ensure that there are healthy bacteria that maintain the balance of the good and bad organisms in the body.

Treatments will be discussed further in the succeeding chapters.

Prevention

Effective prevention includes maintaining a well-balanced diet. You cannot completely get rid of Candida because your body needs it for its normal systemic function, what you need to do is to ensure that the organisms do not multiply in uncontrollable numbers.

Chapter 4 – Natural Treatment for Candida Infection

Natural and alternative medicine practitioners recommend that treatment programs be combined with proper diet and taking supplements. These supplements are to be given gradually so as to avoid the temporary worsening of the symptoms, referred to as "die-off" or Herxheimer reaction, which will be discussed in succeeding chapters. When Candida organisms are killed, their protein fragments and toxins are released that can trigger an antibody response from your immune system. There will be visible improvement of the condition after 2 to 4 weeks.

These are just some of the alternative treatments recommended:

- *Acidophilus* - These bacteria are known to effectively control the growth of Candida. They make the intestinal tract more acidic, thus discouraging the multiplication of Candida at a rapid phase. They also produce hydrogen peroxide that kills Candida on contact.

  Doctors say that taking supplements containing hydrogen peroxide-producing strain of acidophilus, DDS-1, can help reduce the incidence of antibiotic-enhanced Candia growth; in effect, restoring the microbial balance with your digestive tract.

- *Fiber* – Doctors recommend patients to take 1 teaspoon to 1 tablespoon soluble fiber with guar gum, flaxseeds, pectin, or psyllium husks mixed with a glass of water. This should be taken twice a day on an empty stomach.

- *Enteric-coated essential oils* – Enteric-coated capsules have oregano and peppermint oil, plus other volatile oils, that are said to prevent the overgrowth of Candida. Patients are often instructed to take them for several months.

- *Enteric-coated garlic* – Garlic capsules that are enteric-coated are also recommended to prevent Candida from rapidly growing.

- *Grapefruit seed extract* – While this can destroy harmful yeasts and bacteria, it does not destroy the good bacteria.

- *Diet* – Your eating habits are a factor in the rapid growth of Candida in the system. There are certain foods that shouldn't be taken, but there are a group of foods that you can safely eat.

Chapter 5 – Changing Your Diet

Dietary change is an important aspect of Candida infection treatment because yeast tends to dwell in the digestive tract. Basically, there are three food types that you need to reduce intake, if not remove from your diet: sugar, yeasty foods, and fermented foods. However, one of the most glaring symptoms of Candida infection is craving for these foods, particularly the sugary types.

Once you have established that your infection is caused by these foods, it is easier to make the necessary changes in the food you eat. You'll never have a hard time sticking to your menu diet plan if you ask for guidance from a health or nutrition expert.

The environment wherein Candida organisms thrive in is acidic. This acidity actually inhibits your body's ability to absorb vitamins and mineral, and limits the production of enzymes y the digestive proteins. When your body has limited enzymes, you'll having indigestion symptoms, like gas, a feeling of being bloated, increased acidity levels, and become sensitive to certain food types.

Sugar, like fructose (a fruit sugar) feeds on Candida, hence you have to avoid eating or drinking fresh either fresh fruits with high fructose content. Alcohol is also a type of sugar and is a direct food source for Candida Albicans. There are also areas where water undergoes chemical treatment that have health benefits, but for people with Candida infection, water treated with chlorine can make their condition worse. Distilled water is also not a guarantee that bottled water is safe.

What makes the Candida diet difficult is that it can be restrictive. A patient has to muster enough commitment to follow the Candida diet. It is also important to note the general rule that if you have Candida infection, you'll have to be on strict Candida diet for a month for every year that you have the infection. Meaning, if you have had the infection for 10 years, you'll have to follow the strict diet for 10 months.

This is to effectively starve the yeast organisms that are causing the symptoms. You have to understand that the diet is not nutritionally sound and expect not to get the full benefits from the food you eat; hence, you need to take multivitamins and other supplements.

You have to make sure that when you begin to follow the Candida diet, you have to stick with it, but this is what you can look forward to, you can completely treat the infection when you strictly follow the diet.

Something to remember about sugar, there are sugar substitutes and chemical sweeteners that might also make your condition worse, so you'll also have to avoid them. There are, however, natural sweeteners that are derived from plants, which are safer for those who have Candida infection. The perfect example is Vegetable Glycerine that comes from coconut palm. You can get it from health stores and usually come in liquid form, similar to honey, but this is considered to be sweeter.

Foods to Avoid When You Have Candida Infection

- Avoid all kinds of sweets, including those hidden in processed foods, like soups and fruit juices.

- Grains also should be avoided, like prepared flake cereals, including rice, wheat, buckwheat, and corn.

- Make sure that you stay away from granola, instant oats, pearl barley, cornmeal, degerminated microwave popcorn, and blue corn meal. Most people with Candida infection have developed high sensitivity to gluten.

- Pasta is made from flour and water. The flour could be white bread flour or durum flour from semolina. Aside from pasta, you also have to avoid all types of noodles that were made from the same base, including ramen instant noodles, Japanese noodles, and farina.

- Cakes and pastries, doughnuts cookies, and other baked goodies that contain sugar. These include white bread, pita bread, white flour tortillas, and other bread made from wheat.

- Legumes, including peas and beans that contain sweeteners, bean sprouts, fermented tofu called tempeh, tofu, and textured vegetable protein.

- Coconuts, pistachios, walnuts, and peanuts should not be in your diet. Nuts have high amounts of mold which enhances the Candida overgrowth.

- Vegetables, such as potatoes, sweet potatoes, carrots, beets, yams, and parsnips. These are nutrient-dense but they cause Candida overgrowth. They can, however, be re-introduced into your diet in smaller portions gradually.

- Most forms of fruits, whether fresh, dried, canned, or extracts (juiced), have to be avoided. Fruits have high sugar content. Once you have eliminated the infection, you can slowly add fruit into your diet, but make sure they have low sugar contents, like melon, grapefruit, strawberry, and apple.

- Meats and meat products, including pork, cured meat, processed meat, and smoked and packed meats shouldn't be in your diet. Avoid bacon, salami, and sausages. Pork has retroviruses that can survive the cooking process and can be harmful if you have a weakened digestive system. Luncheon meat and other canned meat are loaded with dextrose nitrates, sugars, and sulfates, which can make your symptoms worse.

- All fish types with the exception of wild salmon and sardines. All kinds of shellfish should be avoided. Fish and shellfish have high concentrations of heavy metals and toxins. They will only cause the suppression of your immune system, making you vulnerable to Candida infection.

- Avoid dairy products like cheese, cream, milk, buttermilk, and whey products. Almost all dairy products should be a part of your diet, except for ghee, kefir, probiotic yogurt, and butter. Milk has lactose which is a form of sugar. You can use kefir and yogurt in place of milk because these have undergone the fermentation process wherein lactose has been destroyed.

- Mushrooms and truffles are also to be avoided. While mushrooms do not actually enhance the growth of Candida, but having fungi in your diet can result in inflammatory reaction if you already have Candida infection. Medicinal mushrooms might have a different effect, though.

- Avoid condiments, including ketchup, mayonnaise, regular mustard, horseradish, soy sauce, and relish. Tomato-based sauces have high amounts of hidden sugars, so are condiments and they can aggravate the symptoms so you better not include them in your diet.

- All vinegars, with the exception of apple cider vinegar, are made in a yeast culture. They deplete your stomach with the needed acids. They are also one of the main causes of inflammation in your gut.

- Fats and oils like peanut oil, canola oil, soy oil, and corn oil are contaminated with mold.

- Aside from fruit juices, steer clear of beverages like coffee, black and green tea, energy drinks, and sodas (even the diet or no sugar varieties). Caffeine is known to cause an increase in blood sugar levels, but its main impact is it can cause a weakening of the adrenals and derails proper functionality of your immune system. Coffee has mold. Even decaf would make your condition worse because it still contains residual levels of caffeine.

- Alcohol varieties, such as wine, spirits, beer, liquors, and cider are good for Candida overgrowth. They also cause stress on your immune system.

What Are the Foods that You Can Eat?

When you look at the long list of "forbidden" foods, you might be worried about where you can get your nutrient needs. While it is true that Candida diet actually is low in nutrition, there are still foods that you can eat.

The ideal diet for a person with Candida infection is a high fiber and protein kind of diet, coupled with complex carbohydrates and limited types of fresh fruits. It looks a little something like this:

- 65% high fiber foods (steamed vegetables)
- 20% high protein foods (chicken and eggs)
- 10% complex carbohydrates (rice)
- 5% fresh fruits (those with low sugar contents)

The following is a list of foods that are acceptable if you have Candida infection:

- Grains, but only in moderation. These include amaranth and flour, whole barley, brown basmati rice, texmati brown rice, whole quinoa and flour, cream of rye cereal, wheat berries, unprocessed miler's wheat bran, graham wheat four, saifun (Japanese noodles), whole milet and flour, soba (buckwheat), and udon (Japanese noodles).

- While you have to avoid most known baked products, you can still eat products made from whole grain unsweetened, un-yeasted bread, like capatis, corn chips, unsweetened cakes and crackers, tortillas made from brown, wheat, or corn wheat, and quick breads.

- There are other legumes that you can eat, like dried or frozen black eyed peas, garbanzos, lentils, soybeans, soy flakes, and split peas.

- There are dairy products that are safe to eat even if you have Candida infection. Unsweetened soymilk is okay, so are almond milk, and plain yogurt with acidophilus culture.

- Nuts and seeds like almonds, cashew, hazel, macadamia, Brazil nuts, pine nuts, pecans, pumpkin, sunflower, poppy, and sesame seeds are acceptable.

- You have lime or fresh lemon on some occasions.

- While there are vegetables that shouldn't be part of your diet, there are others that you can still eat, they include Brussels sprouts, broccoli, beans, cabbage, celery, cauliflower, cucumber, green pepper, lettuce, kale, onion, parsley, radish, arugula, spinach, eggplant, and tomatoes.

- There are beverages that you cannot drink, but there are still some that you can, like almond milk, toasted whole barley, unsweetened soy milk, coffee substitute that doesn't have malt, and water (either plain or carbonated).

- When it comes to proteins, you can get your daily supply from chicken, buffalo, deer, duck, elk, eggs, goat, goose, moose, guinea fowl, quail, and turkey.

Antibiotics Might not be a Good Idea

While there are proofs that confirm that Candida overgrowth is brought about by what you eat, there are researches showing the ill effects of taking antibiotics. Prolonged antibiotics intake can enhance the growth of Candida microorganisms, making your infection worse.

How is that? Antibiotics are designed to kill bad bacteria that can cause illnesses and infections. However, antibiotics can also destroy the good bacteria that help regulate the presence of Candida in the body. Prolonged exposure to the potent types of antibiotics can lead to the imbalance of the normal gut flora. This will allow the bad bacteria, parasites, and yeasts to overgrow in your stomach.

How to Protect Yourself from Developing Candida Infection from Antibiotics

Don't take antibiotics until it is necessary. You don't need antibiotics to treat the common cold, sinus infections, or the flu, unless they last for more than 2 weeks or result to extremely high fever.

Let your immune system fight off the most common infections, this is how you will also strengthen your immunity against illnesses. When you take antibiotics at the onset of the most common illnesses, your body will have the tendency to be dependent on antibiotics. This might eventually result to developing your body's resistance to these medications, so, the next time you actually need to take antibiotics, you'll be requiring a higher dosage.

Antibiotics are not also good for children. Kids are still developing and constantly growing, thus they are susceptible to the common viruses. When you let a child take antibiotics to treat the common cold, for instance, his immune system would weaken and do not develop to its full capacity. This will only result in their dependency to antibiotics when they reach adulthood.

There are holistic remedies and alternative treatments for Candida infection and you can read all about them in the succeeding chapters.

Chapter 6 – Home Remedies for Candida Infection

The fact that anybody can develop Candida infection, it is important that everyone is informed about how it can be treated. Aside from changing your diet, there are effective home remedies that can help alleviate the symptoms. There are herb supplements that you can take to help treat the infection.

- Take lactobacillus and bifidus probiotic supplements every day. These bacteria grow in your digestive tract form a protective lining that prevents yeast colonies from forming. For those who have vaginal infections, you can place the probiotic capsules into the vagina before going to bed every night for about two weeks.

  The healthy adult's colon or large intestine should have an estimated 100 trillion good bacteria or 100,000 billion bacteria.

  If you continuously take sufficient amounts of probiotics and lactobacillus and eliminate sugar and yeast from your daily diet, Candida yeast and other "non-friendly" bacteria will not multiply. Since probiotics have no toxic effects, you can take more than the dosage that your doctor told you take.

  The good bacteria that your body has no need for will just be passed in your stools. Doctors often surmise that slight diarrhea is caused by too many good bacteria in your system.

- Taking caprylic acid daily with your meals will help. Caprylic acid is a naturally occurring fatty acid which is recognized to effectively treat Candida infection. It is easily absorbed by the intestines. You need to take a timed-release or enteric-coated form so that it is gradually released throughout your digestive tract.

- Colloidal silver has been used for so many centuries in treating infections. Experts say that it can protect you from up to 650 types of harmful microorganisms and bacteria. Colloidal silver are fine particles of pure silver suspended in water that have active antimicrobial properties. You need it to help eradicate the symptoms of Candida infection. However, you have to make sure that you choose only a high quality silver; otherwise, it can only lead to the unnecessary build up of heavy metal in your body. When this happens, symptoms like the presence of blue fingernails or bluish skin become evident, and these can be permanent.

  Also, using poor quality colloidal silver will kill the probiotics that you have in your intestinal tract. Your doctor would be able to recommend an excellent colloidal silver brand that you can use. Aside from alleviating the symptoms, a good quality colloidal silver product will weaken harmful parasitic organisms, at the same time, boosting your immune system.

While colloidal silver is a potent treatment for Candida infection, it only attacks harmful pathogens, which are anaerobic in nature. It will not destroy the good bacteria, which are aerobic in nature. It does not directly attack the bacteria, but destroys the enzymes that the harmful anaerobic bacteria, yeast, viruses, moulds, and viruses need in order to survive, so you are assured that there is a slim chance of them developing resistance to the treatment. Colloidal silver becomes a catalyst and is not consumed in the process.

Colloidal silver is highly recommended by doctors for these reasons:

- Kills anaerobic bacteria and viruses on contact
- Completely supports your immune system against most types of illnesses and infections
- It can effectively destroy Candida organisms
- Helps accelerate the healing process during injuries and tissue damage

Though its harmful effects are not yet known and proven, this is not recommended for pregnant women.

- Bentonite clay or charcoal is natural clay derived from volcanic ash. It has a variety of smectite minerals and montmorillonite clay. This "edible clay" has been used for over thousands of years; it is also called "healing clay". It is easily absorbed and when taken internally, it assists the intestinal system to get rid of the harmful toxins. The clay will literally pull off the Candida from the intestinal walls. Since the clay itself cannot be absorbed by the body, those unwanted organisms that the clay absorbs are easily passed out with your feces.

  Activated charcoal has also been used for over 2 thousand years and is known to effectively purge harmful toxins and irritants that weaken the digestive tract. It is also highly absorptive.

  Both these supplements can help treat stomach upsets, food poisoning, and travel sickness.

- Psyllium is a seed that is predominant in India, where is it called "isabgol". Its husk is high in fiber content, which is used as laxative and colon cleanser. As psyllium absorbs water it expands and forms a gel, which makes it easier to pass off well-formed stools. Cleansing your colon is an excellent way to rid your body of Candida infection.

- Garlic is known for its potent medicinal properties. It has anti-bacterial and anti-fungal properties that help in the eradication of Candida Albicans. This is an effective home remedy because bacteria and fungi will not develop resistance to garlic, hence, it is easier to purge. Garlic contains allicin, alliinase, and S-allylcysteine, which are effective in fighting off bacteria and fungus.

It is more effective if you eat raw garlic, the only advantage is that raw garlic is pungent and leaves a distinct unpleasant odor on the breath that embarrasses a lot of people.

You might be surprised to find garlic supplements available, so ask your medical practitioner to recommend the best ones for you.

- Green algae, like Chlorella and Spirulina, are often referred to as "green super foods". They grow in warm and alkaline fresh waters all over the world. These are excellent sources of essential amino acids, chelated chemicals, trace minerals, enzymes, and natural plant sugars. They also have rich amounts of calcium, potassium, zinc, manganese, magnesium, selenium, phosphorus, and iron. Also being rich in chlorophyll, they have strong detoxification properties.

  Detoxifying your colon is an effective way of fighting Candida infection because it thrives in toxic environment: take away conducive environment and you get rid of Candida microorganisms.

Chapter 7 – Candida Cleanse in 14 Days

What Is Candida Cleanse?

The best treatment for Candida infection is Candida cleanse. This process helps restore the balance in your system. The main goal of Candida cleansing is to bring Candida down into its normal level since the body also needs this yeast in the system. These are just three of its benefits:

1. Helps your body to maintain the normal balance of colonization of Candida Albicans.
2. Supports and enhances your immune system.
3. Supports your intestinal tract.

A good Candida cleanse is actually dependent on an overall approach that includes Candida diet, which is avoiding foods that feed Candida, and the use of supplements that are anti-fungal to help enhance your digestive system, while successfully cleansing your bowel and lymphatic system and toning your liver.

You'll find a lot of products available in the market that contain fiber that you can safely use to clean out toxins and waste from the body.

There are a variety of ways to do Candida cleanse. There are processes that focus on your liver, kidney, gallbladder, colon, and a lot more. When you decide on doing Candida cleanse, you should first focus on flushing out your colon.

One of the simplest ways to cleanse is to use antifungal supplements for 2 weeks and then switch to probiotics for another 2 weeks. Do this for 3 months.

You need to ensure that your digestive system is also improved since Candida yeast usually feeds on poorly digested food and it will continue to multiply. You'll have to take a course of full spectrum digestive enzymes with each meal for 3 months.

If you are not having bowel movements twice a day and suffering from constipation, you will need to take a mild laxative that will help re-tone the bowel until it improves. You also have to make sure that you add more fiber to your diet, increase water intake, and do regular exercises. Why exercise? It helps your body to work more efficiently and it enhances the detoxification process. Swimming, cycling, and brisk walls would be good exercise routines.

The liver is an integral part of the detoxification process so you have to make sure that it is carrying out its functions effectively. When it cannot handle the high amounts of toxins that it needs to flush out, it will re-absorb the toxins into your system, causing illnesses and infections. Get supplements for your liver, like milk thistle, dandelion root, Vitamin C, and burdock root.

You also have to ensure that you are stressed out because when you become stressed, your body will release sugars into the blood and this will result in Candida overgrowth. Alleviate stress, get massages when you feel you are working too hard or take vacations to unwind, just make sure that your stress level is in check.

The Candida Cleanse

Designing your own good cleanse is not easy, especially considering that most Candida infection sufferers might be experiencing low energy levels and fatigue. This is why most doctors recommend sufferers to eat small portions of salads and vegetables daily throughout the duration of the cleansing process. However, you might want to try a full colon cleanse for 14 days.

- What you can eat

  The diet is almost similar to the standard Candida diet, but it is stricter. To get better results, your diet should consist of raw salads and steamed vegetables only. You don't have to worry, though, since you'll only have this strict regimen for at least 14 days. You might be surprised to find out how your body can easily adjust with this strict diet. When you follow this strict Candida diet, you will end up feeling refreshed, healthy, and light.

  Consider how you have been eating every day and you will realize why it is important for your liver and other internal organs to be given fresh starts. Unhealthy eating is downright not beneficial for your body. For example, fast foods have additives, most of the beef have growth hormones added, and most fish schools get chemicals because of unscrupulous individuals who pollute the oceans. When you minimize on these, you also reduce the toxins, so the best thing to do is to eat fresh produce to jumpstart the cleansing process.

  However, not all vegetables would be suitable for you, make sure you stay away from starchy veggies, like potatoes, sweet potatoes, yams, winter wash, and corn. You'll be surprised the versatility that you can create in your meals in just the 2-week period of Candida cleanse. You'll have a variety of dishes that you can create just by adding the most basic flavorings to your salads and veggies, like salt and pepper, lemon juice, herbs, and spices.

  If you want to up it up a little bit, you can go on a "liquid-only-cleanse". Two to three bowls of vegetable a day would be a good alternative. Your vegetable broth would be able to help replace the depleted minerals that you body needs. If you think you cannot commit to the liquid-only-cleanse for two weeks, you can still try it for the last two days of your Candida cleanse.

- What you can drink

  The most important thing is you increase your water intake during the cleansing process. This way, you can give your body the best chances of expelling as many toxins as possible. Water will keep your digestive system functioning as it should and it accelerates the purging process.

  Detoxifying drinks would also help because these drinks are designed to support the liver, facilitate bowel movements, and condition your body to eject Candida toxins rapidly.

  Earlier, bentonite clay was mentioned, it doesn't mix well with water so doctors recommend that you buy its liquid form that has been made available today. You can easily add it to your fiber supplement and mix in a blender and drink. Once consumed, you have to drink a glass of water. Bentonite absorbs the toxins and fiber will flush it out of your system via the colon. Just to keep in mind to drink this on an empty stomach and you are not to eat anything an hour before and after. Do this 2 to 3 times a day.

Why You Need to Do Colon Cleanse

With today's modern lifestyle, your colon is subjected to a lot of stress. Think about the amount of fast food staples you have eaten in the past, how many times you have taken prescription drugs for common illnesses, or the alcoholic beverages you have consumed; all these keep your colon working harder than it should. Then add to that having Candida overgrowth and you have an unhealthy and stressed colon.

Your colon is like your waste pipe. The moment all the nutrients have been absorbed and processed the waste that come from the food you ate will pass through your colon and get flushed out from your body. However, it is possible that feces, including Candida yeast colonies, can get backed up and solidified in your colon. Needless to say, if you don't do regular colon cleansing, these formations will be trapped in there for a long time. This will result in the slow release of harmful toxins into your system.

The waste matter will eventually harden and will be fixated into the walls of your colon. This can cause the feeling of bloating. What's worse is that this waste material is the perfect breeding ground for Candida yeast, and you risk the release of toxins into your bloodstream. Bottom line is, you need to flush them out of your system and you can only do that with an effective colon cleanse process.

Colonic Irrigation

Colonic irrigation is a process that can make the cleansing process more effective. This will accelerate the loosening of the hardened fecal matter in the colon and eventually expel them, including Candida yeast and its byproducts. However, if you are not suffering from constipation, this is not recommended for you. The drawback to this process is that it removes too much of the "friendly" bacteria in your gut, in addition to removing Candida yeast. Make sure that your doctor recommends that you do this process along with your Candida diet.

This is a treatment that needs the help of a colonic expert because a plastic tube will have to be inserted into your rectum where warm water will be passed into your colon. Before insertion, you will first be massage in your lower stomach area to help loosen the hardened matter so that it will be easier for you colon to expunge them.

Is Colon (Candida) Cleansing Safe?

Cleansing is a healthy and safe way to "reset" your health. It boosts the functions of your liver and colon and it will help detoxify your body. However, this is not recommended for those with major health conditions. The best thing to do is to consult with a health practitioner for any of your concerns, whether they are minor or major. It is important that before you subject your body to any kind of treatment, you have all the information you need about the procedure and possible side effects.

7 Key Factors to Remember

Here is a list of the 7 most important key points to remember during the Candida cleanse period:

- The role of yeast

  The Candida diet was designed to simply purge out all the harmful toxins and fungi that contaminate your digestive tract. Cleansing can effectively remove excess yeast from the body by cutting down on your food consumption, especially those that cause Candida overgrowth.

  It has been recommended that you reduce on the food that contains yeasts. In most cases it is useful because most foods that are made with yeast also have high sugar or starch content. While you do not want to eat too much yeast so as not to boost Candida yeast's overgrowth, you cannot stress yourself out thinking whether the bread you are eating has yeast or not. The key phrase should be, "everything in moderation".

- Restrictions on carbohydrate intake

  It is recommended that you eat food that has low carbohydrate-content, like chicken, turkey meat, and non-starchy vegetables. It is recommended that you consume less than 60% of carbohydrates in your diet for the first week of your Candida cleanse.

- Fermented foods

Fermented foods have sugar and starch, thus they are the best food source for the fungus. Mushrooms, beers, and tomato paste have to be reduced, if not completely eliminated from your diet.

- The role of natural yogurt

To speed up the process, you have to add yogurt in your diet. It is an excellent and natural source of lactobacillus acidophilus, which is good for your immune system.

- The anti-Candida diet and protein

Candida diet allows you to eat protein, but not too much, lest you want to congest the system. Fish is highly recommended, steamed fish in particular. Eggs would also be good and eggs are easy to digest. But remember to eat the egg raw, or you can mix them with a little bit of fresh milk if you can't stand the taste of raw eggs.

- Taking supplements

It is important that you take supplements in addition to Candida diet because diet alone will not remove Candida microorganisms completely. You have been given a thorough discussion about supplements in the previous chapters.

- This is not a miracle diet

Keep in mind that this is a process. You don't treat Candida infection in a jiffy, it takes time and you have to be patient and fully committed when you decide to follow the strict Candida diet. The 14-day Candida cleanse that you choose is just the minimum, the doctor might recommend a longer period if the infection is not fully treated in that short amount of time.

Lots of sufferers struggle because the diet itself is hard to follow. How can a person survive with very limited food choices? But what is important that you fully commit to what you want to achieve and you will be successful in time.

Candida Cleanse Tips for Success

1. Remember to check the ingredients of anything you buy at the grocery store. It pays to read the labels knowing that Candida diet has a lot of restrictions.

2. Using organic vanilla extract could be a good choice when you need to cook with vanilla extract. It doesn't contain sugar. It is different from regular vanilla extract which has sugar.

3. Garlic is an excellent counter-measure for Candida. It does work wonders if you chop or crush several cloves and let them sit for 15 minutes before continue using them for cooking. Garlic is also good for salads, fish, and meat dishes.

4. Cinnamon is good at preventing Candida overgrowth and preventing inflammation. It effectively inhibits yeast growth and is an excellent source of fiber, iron, manganese, and calcium. Did you know that just by smelling cinnamon, you already improve your concentration and memory? It also helps stabilize blood sugar levels. It adds flavors to vegetables, and chicken dishes.

5. Nutmeg helps relieve bloating brought about by Candida infection. It is also a good antibacterial agent and effectively kills the bad bacteria found in your mouth and throat. It also helps in cleansing and detoxifying the liver and the kidneys. It is rich in Vitamin B-complex.

6. Fresh ginger helps in the detoxification process.

7. You can use the sweetener xylitol as alternative to sugar. It has long been proven to be a good anti-fungal agent and it effectively inhibits the growth of Candida yeast. However, be sure not to use the corn-based version.

8. Unflavored yogurt helps enhance the growth of good bacteria in your colon. It is also an excellent source of calcium. Calcium inhibits the excess growth of the cells in the lining of the colon.

9. If you are tired of drinking unflavored water, you can try squeezing lemon or lime juice into the water you drink as this adds flavor, at the same time enhancing the water's ability to flush out toxins. It also helps increase hydration.

10. Cleansing with peppermint tea and ginger tea would also help flush out dead yeasts from the system; thus preventing Candida die-off. Die-off will be discussed in the next chapter.

Chapter 8 – Candida Die-Off

Die-off is the term used to describe the mass death of pathogenic organisms inhabiting the body. This phenomenon creates numerous symptoms.

What Is Candida Die-Off?

When you have Candida infection, it is vital in your full recovery that the yeast population is reduced to normal levels, or even to below normal levels for susceptible individuals. You have learned in the previous chapters that you can treat Candida infection by doing Candida cleanse that follows a strict Candida diet. Living yeast causes the different symptoms by releasing toxic metabolic byproducts into your body, essentially, if you kill these yeasts, they will release larger amounts of these harmful toxins.

It would take time for the body to sluice these toxins, especially if there are a huge number of yeast cells that die at one time. Keep in mind, as well, that these dead yeast cells have to be eliminated. The release toxins will be in your bloodstream and can affect the functions of your internal organs including your kidneys, liver, colon, and lymph, as they make their way out of your body.

In most cases, sufferers who experience Candida die-off complain that their existing Candida infection symptoms worsen to greater extents.

Feeling that your symptoms and condition worsen even after following the strict diet and cleansing process could be quite alarming in the beginning. However, it is still encouraging to know that this more than confirms the presence of Candida and its susceptibility to the anti-fungal treatment you are using.

No two individual experience the same symptoms of Candida die-off during their recovery period. Though there is a surefire way to pre-determine at what point or degree an individual is likely to feel it.

Some sufferers begin the cleansing process and see improvements almost immediately, citing positive effects like better bowel movements and increased energy. These are the ones whose Candida die-off experience is still likely to occur, but it would take a few more weeks until the onset of the symptoms.

For others who feel worse right after initializing treatment may feel worst almost immediately as a response to temporary toxicity. Sufferers might suffer from flu-like symptoms, numbness, skin rashes, vaginal irritation and discharge, fatigue, constipation, diarrhea, or fatigue.

The die-off reaction usually lasts from one day to a week and likely to come during the duration of the program. Experts say that it is likely to occur during the first week. But as your body gains back its strength, your body's susceptibility to Candida toxins would be reduced, and die-off symptoms would also be alleviated.

The severity of the symptoms will depend on how weak or strong the organs affected by Candida yeast are, the strength of your body's immune system, the degree of the infection, and the emotional and even the environmental stress you are having. There are also different approaches to treating the symptoms. It is important for sufferers to know their body well so that they will also know what treatment and approach would be appropriate. They shouldn't attempt to rush the progress because they will only experience more severe reactions.

Managing Candida Die-Off

Candida yeast commonly inhabits the walls of the colon. It usually thrives behind and inside any build-up of fecal waste. If there is a large amount of fecal build-up or intestinal mucous, the occurrence of die-off is delayed or prolonged. You will need a longer period of cleansing and strict dieting to completely eliminate the wastes so that the anti-fungal agents are able to fully function.

Having mentioned this, your body's response to the cleansing process should become noticeable after a few weeks. Some people become too impatient to feel the die-off symptoms in order to confirm how the process is progressing.

Remember this the moment you begin feeling the die-off symptoms, you'll need to reduce the dosage of your anti-fungal agent a bit and gradually increase it as your body copes with the sudden rush of detoxification challenges.

Of course, you would want to prevent die-off symptoms from manifesting during the cleansing process. Thing is, more die-off symptoms do not really indicate that you are eliminating more yeast; it could be that the eliminative organs are just becoming overwhelmed. This should be a cause for alarm because when this happens, die-off becomes an adversary instead of a friend. If your body is overwhelmed and stressed, it can derail the healing process.

What you want is a slow and gradual process of purging of the Candida yeast from the body; it is healthier and more effective.

The best thing to do is to take the anti-fungal agent, beginning with a lower dose and gradually increasing as you progress and your body responds accordingly. If you are experiencing moderate to severe die-off symptoms, you will need to cut back on the dosage to reduce the number of dead yeast cells.

Die-Off Symptoms

Symptoms vary for each sufferer since each one has different degrees of Candida infestation. Your liver is the main pathway where toxin elimination happens. When die-off symptoms manifest, that would mean that your liver is overwhelmed.

These are just some of the symptoms that you might experience during die-off. (Die-off is also referred to by experts as, Herxheimer reaction.)

- Nausea and vomiting

- Fatigue, headache dizziness

- Bloating

- Constipation or diarrhea

- Gas

- Swollen glands

- Joint and muscle pain

- Increased heart rate

- Chills

- Cold feeling in the extremities

- Heavy sweating

- Fever

- Breakouts on skin

- Recurring prostate and vaginal infections

- Recurring sinus infections

How to Cope with Candida Die-Off

Symptoms would normally clear up in a week, but there are cases when they last longer. Here are just some of the things that you can do to minimize the reaction or to fast track the elimination of the toxins:

- Make sure that you take supplements that will help in the eradication of the toxins. A good supplement should be able to convert neurotoxin acetaldehyde into acetic acid, which will be removed from the body; it can also be converted into some useful digestive enzymes.

- Temporarily discontinue taking your anti-fungal supplements. Anti-fungal agents break down the walls of the Candida yeast cells, wherein they will release the harmful toxins that Candida produces. When you reduce or discontinue the supplements, the amount of toxins that are released into your bloodstream will greatly be reduced. When die-off symptoms are gone, you can begin to increase the dosage again.

- Reduce probiotics. These do not necessarily cause die-off symptoms but if you begin to experience the symptoms, you also have to reduce the dosage even for a short while or until the die-off systems are not manifested anymore.

- Increase water intake. Drinking water is the most natural way to flush out harmful toxins. Further increasing your intake would ensure that toxins will be washed down at a rapid phase.

- Take a rest. When you are stressed at work or at home, you need to take rests and slow down from your fast paced lifestyle. As you very well know now, stress can be a cause of weakening your body, particularly the adrenals, which will result in your body's inability to fight off harmful pathogens. Boost your immune system when you relax and take some time off.

- Try other detoxification methods like brushing and sauna.

- Increase Vitamin C dosage and take twice a day.

Chapter 9 – Preventing Recurrent Candida Infection

Just when you thought your Candida Albicans infection is gone, you begin to feel the symptoms again - vaginal itching, burning sensation, and discharge, and a host of other symptoms. You might be suffering from recurrent Candida infection and you have to consult with your doctor immediately.

It doesn't matter if the symptoms turn up in a week's time or in the cases of some people that the symptoms begin to manifest again months after the treatment. This can be a frustrating occurrence.

Why Recurrence Might Happen

There are a lot of possible reasons on the recurrence of Candida infection. One of the most basic ones is that yeast thrives in warm and moist conditions; in this case, the vagina has these conditions. Most of the time, a recurrence is more likely to manifest in the vagina because of those factors. It is further aggravated if you wear synthetic underwear or you are used to wearing tight jeans. These materials do not let the genital area "breathe" so it stays moist and warm all the time, the perfect breeding ground for bacteria.

Here are some additional factors that contribute to the recurrence of Candida infection in the vagina:

- Changes in the immune system that can lead to the changes in the pH of the vagina.

- When a woman gets regular heavy periods, it results to more blood in the area, thus making it conducive for bacteria to grow.

- Tears in the vagina and irritation brought about by inadequate lubrication during sex. These tears make the vagina more prone to infection.

- The presence of underlying tissues, like diabetes, that put a lot of women at greater risk of infection, especially Candida infection.

- Smoking compromises the immune system, and this makes one vulnerable to infections.

- Women who have been treated for a different disease, and who had to take antibiotics are put at greater risk of recurring Candida infection.

- Untreated diabetes can lead to increased sugar levels in the blood and urine, and you have learned in the previous chapters that excess sugar can contribute to Candida overgrowth. If you have just completed treatment for Candida infection and you are not aware that you are suffering from diabetes, it puts you at higher risk.

- Pregnancy and other hormonal disorders can also bring about recurrent Candida infection in the vagina.

Symptoms

When there is a re-growth of fungus in your vagina, symptoms will become visible: thick, cottage cheese-like discharge, and persistent itching. Women who frequently have recurring Candida infection are at high risk because of a few reasons.

Avoid Recurrence

Since one of the main reasons why a recurrence happens in the vagina is the condition of the area, here are some tips to ensure that the infection doesn't recur:

- If you are used to wearing synthetic panties, you might need to switch to cotton. Cotton is more suited for the skin and it absorbs moisture too.

- You can wear pajama bottoms and you can go bare instead, this will allow for better air circulation to the genital area as you sleep.

- If you usually wear spandex and tight jeans, try switching to more breathable and comfortable materials.

- Make sure that you wipe dry the genital area after using the toilet.

- Take antibiotics only when it is absolutely needed and directed by your doctor.

- Do not attempt to douche your genitals. While you might have heard about the benefits of vaginal douching, it causes more damage than good, as verified by most doctors themselves.

- Do not engage in sexual intercourse until you are sure that the infection has been completely treated.

- During your menstrual periods, change pads and tampons frequently. This is good for hygiene and keeps the vagina moisture-free.

If you continue experiencing the symptoms after making a few changes, you might need to ask your doctor to rule out other possible medical conditions. This enables you to get the proper treatment for your illness.

There are some women who are more susceptible to Candida yeast infections because of poor hygiene habits and unhealthy eating.

Getting a Proper Diagnosis

Since you have had the infection before, you might opt to self-medicate and use over-the-counter drugs and supplements to treat the infection. However, it is imperative that you consult with your doctor because there might be more serious illnesses that should be properly diagnosed. A sexually transmitted disease almost has the same symptoms as Candida yeast infection.

Getting an accurate diagnosis is important. You have to make sure that the underlying causes and symptoms are dealt with accordingly.

The Three-Step Prevention of Recurrence

Candida yeast infection is quite common among women who are of childbearing age. When a recurrence occurs, you have to work closely with your doctor to ensure that the condition doesn't recur.

Step #1 – Look at the Environmental Factors

1. Keep your genital area clean and dry to discourage Candida overgrowth.

   - Don't wear pantyhose.

   - Change your wet swimsuit immediately after swimming.

   - Change to fresh underwear before going to bed.

2. Avoid using scented soaps, detergents, and other personal hygiene products.

   - Do not use scented toilet paper. This can cause irritation on your vagina that can trigger the growth of Candida Albicans.

   - Switch to eco-friendly laundry detergents and fabric softeners. You might even want to skip fabric softeners all-together.

   - Avoid scented sanitary pads, panty liners, and tampons.

   - Wash the vagina with gentle cleanser. Keep in mind that you cannot use antibacterial soaps because these can alter the pH balance in your vagina, making it vulnerable to infection.

3. Have your partner use condoms without spermicide if you experience irritation during sex. There are women who are sensitive to spermicide and repeated use of these types of condoms can lead to irritation and Candida infection.

4. Ask your partner to be tested or seek treatment for infections if you notice a recurrence of your condition.

- Better speak to your doctor. While Candida infection is not transmitted through sexual intercourse, there are doctors who would recommend that sex partners get tested if one person is showing symptoms of an infection.

- Abstain from sex if you have the infection.

5. You might need to change your hormonal birth control pill if you repeatedly suffer from Candida infection. Consult your medical practitioner about it.

Step #2 – Dietary Concerns

1. Add milk products with acidophilus to your diet.

2. Reduce sugar on your diet.

Without enumerating them all over again, you will have to do Candida cleansing and follow a strict Candida diet all over again.

Step #3 – Address Possible Underlying Factors and Conditions

1. Consult with your doctor if you are experiencing recurring Candida infections and you are suffering from diabetes, lupus, HIV, or other illnesses that affect the immune system. There might be underlying causes that results in the recurrence of your infection.

2. Discuss possible treatment strategies that would control the symptoms and completely prevent and treat the infection.

3. Strictly follow instructions and prescriptions by your doctor to ensure that the infection doesn't recur.

What if the Treatment Does not Work?

If the treatment doesn't work and the condition recurs, these might be the possible reasons:

- Your condition might have been misdiagnosed. If you can consult another medical practitioner and get a second opinion for your condition, it would be better. You need proper diagnosis so appropriate treatment can be done.

- You might not have strictly followed the Candida diet.

- You might have had to treat an illness after you have completed your Candida infection treatment. If you needed to take antibiotics to treat a specific illness, this might be the reason why your Candida infection recurred.

Candida Albicans infection has a lot of facets. There are a lot of things to learn about it in order to give proper diagnosis and appropriate treatment to the patients. It is a condition that needs strict compliance and commitment to the treatments in order to completely treat the condition and prevent recurrence.

Conclusion

Thank you again for downloading this book!

I hope you enjoyed reading about my book on

    Finally, if you enjoyed this book, please take the time to share your thoughts and It'd be greatly appreciated!

Thank you!

www.ingramcontent.com/pod-product-compliance
Lightning Source LLC
Chambersburg PA
CBHW081803280526
45789CB00008B/2979